GESTATIONAL DIABETES COOKBOOK

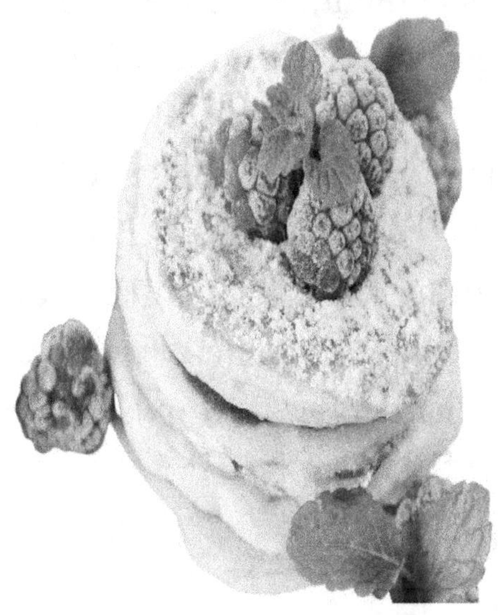

The Healthy, Tasty, Recipes for Gestational Diabetes

Anita Mark

Table of contents

Chapter 1

Introduction

Gestational diabetes is a kind of condition that affects some women during pregnancy. It is a form of diabetes that develops during pregnancy and typically resolves after childbirth. The condition is characterized by high blood sugar levels that can cause complications for both the mother and the developing fetus.

The cause of gestational diabetes is not fully understood, but it is believed to be related to hormonal changes that occur during pregnancy. As the placenta grows, it produces hormones that can interfere with the body's ability to use insulin effectively, leading to insulin resistance and high blood sugar levels.

Women who are at higher risk for gestational diabetes include those who are overweight or obese, have a family history of diabetes, have previously given birth to a baby weighing more than 9 pounds, or have had gestational diabetes in a previous pregnancy.

The symptoms of gestational diabetes can be mild or nonexistent, which is why it is often detected through routine prenatal screening. If left untreated, gestational diabetes can increase the risk of complications during pregnancy and childbirth, including preeclampsia, preterm birth, and cesarean delivery.

To diagnose gestational diabetes, a woman will typically undergo a glucose screening test between 24 and 28 weeks of pregnancy. This test involves drinking a sugary solution and having blood drawn to measure blood sugar levels. If the results of the screening test are abnormal, a woman will undergo a more extensive glucose tolerance test to confirm the diagnosis.

The treatment for gestational diabetes usually involves making dietary changes, increasing physical activity, and monitoring blood sugar levels. Women with gestational diabetes are often advised to follow a balanced meal plan that includes a variety of nutrient-dense foods, with a focus on whole grains, fruits, vegetables, lean proteins, and healthy fats. Portion control is also important, as consuming too many carbohydrates at once can cause blood sugar levels to spike.

Exercise can help lower blood sugar levels and improve insulin sensitivity. Women with gestational diabetes are often advised to engage in moderate-intensity exercise for at least 30 minutes a day, most days of the week. Examples of suitable exercises include walking, swimming, and prenatal yoga.

Monitoring blood sugar levels is an essential part of managing gestational diabetes. Women with gestational diabetes may be asked to check their blood sugar levels multiple times a day and keep a log of their readings. If blood sugar levels cannot be controlled through diet and exercise alone, insulin therapy may be necessary.

In conclusion, gestational diabetes is a form of diabetes that develops during pregnancy and typically resolves after childbirth. The condition is characterized by high blood sugar levels and can cause complications for both the mother and the developing fetus. Treatment typically involves making dietary changes, increasing physical activity, and monitoring blood sugar levels. Early diagnosis and effective management can help ensure a healthy pregnancy and childbirth.

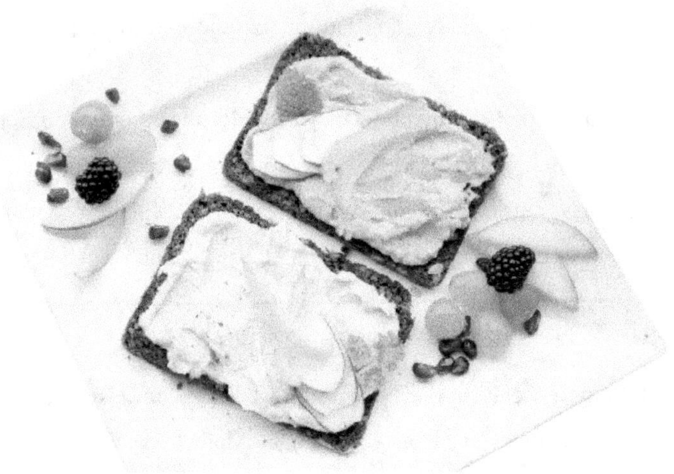

Significance of eating nutritious food during pregnancy

Eating a healthy, balanced diet during pregnancy is essential for the health and well-being of both the mother and the developing fetus. Pregnancy is a time of increased nutritional needs, and a woman's diet plays a crucial role in ensuring that these needs are met.

A healthy diet during pregnancy provides the essential nutrients that the developing fetus needs to grow and develop properly. This includes nutrients such as folic acid, iron, calcium, and protein, which are all important for the development of the fetal brain, bones, and organs.

Eating a healthy diet during pregnancy can also help prevent complications such as gestational diabetes and preeclampsia. Gestational diabetes is a form of diabetes that develops during pregnancy and can cause complications for both the mother and the fetus. Preeclampsia is a potentially serious condition that can cause high blood pressure, protein in the urine, and other complications.

In addition to preventing complications, eating a healthy diet during pregnancy can also help women maintain a healthy weight.

Excessive weight gain during pregnancy can increase the risk of complications such as preterm birth, cesarean delivery, and gestational diabetes.

Furthermore, a healthy diet during pregnancy can help ensure that the mother has the energy and nutrients needed to support the growth and development of the fetus, while also meeting her own increased nutritional needs. This can help prevent fatigue and other symptoms associated with pregnancy.

To ensure a healthy diet during pregnancy, women should focus on consuming a variety of nutrient-dense foods. This includes whole grains, fruits, vegetables, lean proteins, and healthy fats. Foods that are high in sugar, saturated fat, and sodium should be consumed in moderation.

Pregnant women should also be mindful of their calorie intake, as the body's energy needs increase during pregnancy. However, this does not necessarily mean that women need to eat significantly more food than they did before pregnancy. The amount of additional calories needed will depend on factors such as pre-pregnancy weight, age, and activity level.

In addition to eating a healthy diet, pregnant women should also stay hydrated by drinking plenty of water and other fluids throughout the day. Adequate hydration is essential for maintaining healthy blood flow and helping the body eliminate waste products.

Overall, eating a healthy, balanced diet during pregnancy is essential for the health and well-being of both the mother and the developing fetus. It can help prevent complications, promote healthy weight gain, and provide the essential nutrients needed for fetal growth and development. Pregnant women should focus on consuming a variety of nutrient-dense foods, staying hydrated, and being mindful of their calorie intake. Consultation with a healthcare provider or registered dietitian can help pregnant women develop a healthy meal plan tailored to their individual needs.

An Overview of the Cookbook

The complete gestational diabetes cookbook offers guidance on healthy nutrition for expectant mothers who have been diagnosed with the condition. The cookbook is designed to assist pregnant women in controlling their blood sugar levels and avoiding difficulties.

The cookbook contains a selection of nutrient-rich dishes that are created to fulfill the special dietary requirements of pregnant women with gestational diabetes. The recipes employ straightforward ingredients that are simple to locate at the grocery store and are created to be simple to prepare.

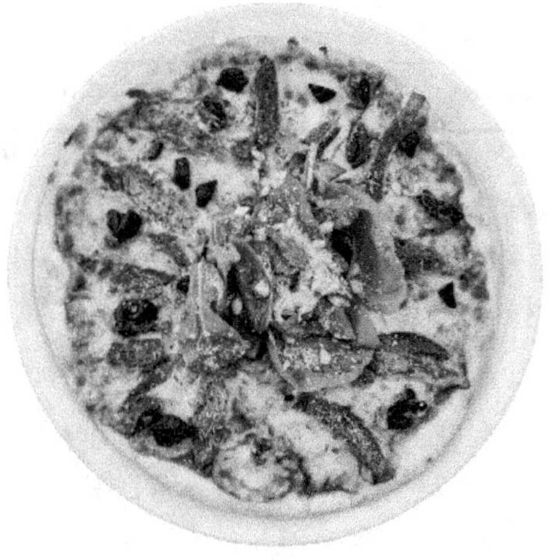

The cookbook for gestational diabetes emphasizes whole grains, fruits, vegetables, lean meats, and healthy fats in its meals. Additionally, the cookbook offers guidance on meal preparation, portion control, and blood sugar control.

The cookbook also offers advice on regulating blood sugar levels, the dangers of gestational diabetes, and the significance of eating healthfully throughout pregnancy. The cookbook is intended to be a useful tool for pregnant women with gestational diabetes who might have trouble organizing and preparing meals.

Women who have been diagnosed with gestational diabetes and are searching for advice on healthy nutrition throughout pregnancy might benefit from using the gestational diabetes cookbook. The cookbook offers a selection of nutrient-rich dishes that are designed to satisfy the special dietary requirements of pregnant women with gestational diabetes. Additionally, the cookbook offers guidance on meal preparation, portion control, and blood sugar control.

Overall, for women who have been diagnosed with gestational diabetes and are searching for helpful advice on healthy nutrition throughout pregnancy, the gestational diabetes cookbook is a great resource. The cookbook has a selection of delectable, nutrient-dense dishes that are specially adapted to address the special dietary demands of pregnant women with gestational diabetes. It is simple to use. Women with gestational diabetes can ensure a safe pregnancy and lower their risk of difficulties for both themselves and their growing fetus by adhering to the cookbook's advice.

Chapter 2

Meaning of Gestational diabetes and causes.

A kind of diabetes called gestational diabetes mellitus (GDM) appears during pregnancy. It happens when the hormone that controls blood sugar levels, insulin, cannot be produced or used by the body as intended. This leads to elevated blood sugar levels, which can have several negative effects on the mother and the fetus as it develops.

Although the exact causes of gestational diabetes are unknown, it is thought that they are linked to the hormonal changes that take place during pregnancy. It may become more challenging for the body to adequately manufacture or use insulin as a result of these hormonal changes.

Being overweight or obese, having a family history of diabetes, being older than 25, having previously given birth to a child weighing more than 9 pounds, and having gestational diabetes in a prior pregnancy are risk factors for gestational diabetes.

Polycystic ovarian syndrome (PCOS), a history of gestational diabetes in a prior pregnancy, and other medical disorders including hypertension or high cholesterol are additional variables that may raise the chance of developing gestational diabetes.

There are a variety of possible concerns associated with gestational diabetes for both the mother and the growing fetus. These include premature labor and delivery, an increased chance of developing type 2 diabetes later in life, and pre-eclampsia, a dangerous illness marked by high blood pressure and protein in the urine.

Along with these issues, gestational diabetes can raise the likelihood that the growing fetus will experience other health issues like macrosomia (excessive fetal growth), hypoglycemia (low blood sugar), and respiratory distress syndrome (a condition where the lungs are not fully formed).

Dietary adjustments, physical activity, and any necessary medication are often combined to manage gestational diabetes. A nutritious, balanced diet high in whole grains, fruits, vegetables, lean meats, and healthy fats is advocated for women with gestational diabetes. Additionally, meals that are heavy in salt, saturated fat, and sugar should be avoided.

Exercise can help increase insulin sensitivity and reduce blood sugar levels, making it a crucial part of controlling gestational diabetes.

Most days of the week, moderate-intensity exercise is recommended for women with gestational diabetes for at least 30 minutes each day.

To assist control blood sugar levels, medication may be necessary in some circumstances. This might involve taking oral medicines like metformin or insulin injections.

Overall, gestational diabetes is a dangerous illness with a variety of possible side effects for both the mother and the growing fetus. However, women with gestational diabetes can have good pregnancies and birth healthy infants with the right treatment. To secure the greatest results for themselves and their unborn children, it is crucial for women who are at risk of gestational diabetes to obtain regular prenatal care and follow the advice of their healthcare experts.

Gestational diabetes's risks.

During pregnancy, gestational diabetes mellitus (GDM), a type of diabetes, develops. It takes place when the body is unable to create enough insulin or utilize it as it should. Insulin regulates blood sugar levels. If it is not effectively managed, gestational diabetes can have several negative effects on both the mother and the developing fetus.

Mother-related issues:

Two signs of the hazardous condition of preeclampsia are high blood pressure and protein in the urine. Pregnant women with gestational diabetes are more prone to develop preeclampsia.

Women with gestational diabetes are more likely to experience complications that call for cesarean delivery, such as fetal distress, macrosomia, or other issues.

Developing type 2 diabetes risk: Type 2 diabetes in later life is more likely to strike women who had gestational diabetes during pregnancy.

Hypoglycemia: Low blood sugar levels may occur as a result of improper blood sugar management. This might have side effects including weakness, dizziness, and confusion.

difficulties for the fetus throughout development:

Macrosomia: Pregnancy-related diabetes may result in an abnormal amount of fetal growth, which may lead to macrosomia, a condition in which the infant is larger than average. The likelihood of birth problems including shoulder dystocia and the need for a cesarean delivery are both increased by macrosomia.

Hypoglycemia: A developing fetus may experience seizures and breathing problems as a result of low blood sugar levels.

Respiratory distress syndrome (RDS), a condition where the lungs are still developing, is more likely to affect newborns whose mothers have gestational diabetes.

Jaundice: Babies delivered to mothers with gestational diabetes may be more susceptible to developing jaundice, a condition in which a buildup of bilirubin results in the skin and eye whites appearing yellow.

Overall, gestational diabetes should be carefully treated to prevent any potential negative effects on the mother or the developing fetus. Pregnant women with gestational diabetes should have normal prenatal care and strict medical supervision to control their blood sugar levels and reduce the likelihood of complications. This could require making dietary changes, working out often, and, in some cases, taking medication to manage blood sugar levels. Gestational diabetic women may also require further testing, such as fetal monitoring and ultrasounds, to ensure the health of the developing fetus. However, with the aid of proper management, the majority of pregnant women with gestational diabetes can have successful pregnancies and give birth to healthy children.

Pregnant women are susceptible to a kind of diabetes known as gestational diabetes mellitus (GDM). When the body cannot properly produce or use insulin, high blood sugar levels occur. If gestational diabetes is not managed, there are several risks for both the mother and the developing fetus.

Macronutrients needed (carbohydrates, protein, and fat).

Carbohydrates, proteins, and fats are the three primary nutrients that the body needs in considerable amounts and are referred to as macronutrients. Each macronutrient has a specific function in the body, therefore it's critical to eat the correct kinds of amounts of them to be healthy.

Carbohydrates: The body's main source of energy is carbohydrate-based. They are converted into glucose, which the body uses as fuel in the cells. While all carbs are necessary for the body to operate, not all carbohydrates are the same. Simple carbs, including those in sugar and processed meals, can raise blood sugar levels and contribute to weight gain. Complex carbs, such as those in whole grains, fruits, and vegetables, give you a consistent stream of energy and are crucial for eating a balanced diet.

Depending on parameters including age, sex, and level of physical activity, different amounts of carbs are suggested daily. Typically, 45–65 percent of daily calories should come from carbs.

Protein: The creation and repair of bodily tissues depend on protein. It is also important for the body to produce the hormones, enzymes, and other chemicals that are required for optimal bodily operation. Meat, fish, eggs, beans, and nuts are examples of foods that contain protein.

Depending on parameters including age, sex, and level of physical activity, different amounts of protein are suggested daily. Adults should typically ingest 0.8 grams of protein for every kilogram of body weight per day.

Fat: Fat is necessary for a variety of body processes, such as the hormone synthesis process, the absorption of vitamins, and the protection of organs. All fats are not created equal, though. Unsaturated fats have the potential to improve health whereas saturated and trans fats can raise the risk of heart disease.

Various factors, including age, sex, and amount of physical activity, affect the required daily consumption of fat. Unsaturated fats, including those in nuts, seeds, and avocados, should make up the majority of the 20–35% of daily calories that come from fat.

It is crucial to remember that each person's requirements for specific macronutrients may vary depending on their activity level, age, gender, and health status. An individual's macronutrient requirements can be ascertained and a customized nutrition plan can be created by speaking with a healthcare professional or registered dietitian.

As a result, macronutrients are crucial for preserving healthy health. Protein is vital for creating and repairing tissues, carbohydrates provide the body with energy, and fat is required for numerous biological processes. For maintaining a balanced diet and preventing chronic illnesses, consuming these macronutrients in the correct proportions is crucial. People can satisfy their nutritional demands and attain optimal health by eating a range of healthy foods from each macronutrient category.

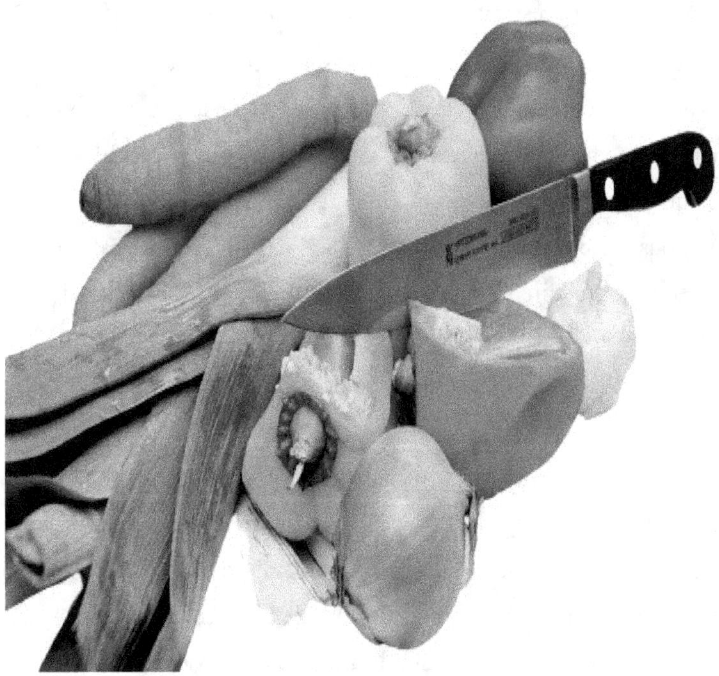

Chapter 3

Glycemic Index and Glycemic Load

According to how rapidly they cause blood sugar levels to rise after consumption, carbohydrates are ranked on the glycemic index (GI). The amount and type of carbohydrates in a food are considered when calculating the glycemic load (GL). Managing blood sugar levels and avoiding chronic illnesses like type 2 diabetes may need an understanding of the glycemic index and glycemic load.

On a scale of 0-100, the glycemic index assesses carbohydrates; pure glucose receives a score of 100. Foods having a high glycemic index digest and absorb fast, which causes a sharp increase in blood sugar levels. White bread, white rice, and sweetened beverages are a few examples of high-GI foods. Low glycemic index foods take longer to digest and absorb, gradually raising blood sugar levels. Whole grains, fruits, and vegetables are among the foods that have a low GI.

The glycemic load considers both the kind and amount of carbohydrates in a dish. It is computed by dividing by 100 after calculating the food's glycemic index by the number of carbs in a serving. Inferring how food will impact blood sugar levels in this way provides a more realistic picture. those having a high glycemic load can cause blood sugar levels to increase quickly, whereas those with a low glycemic load are less likely to do so.

Managing blood sugar levels and avoiding chronic illnesses like type 2 diabetes may need an understanding of the glycemic index and glycemic load. Obesity, type 2 diabetes, and heart disease have all been associated with diets heavy in high GI and high GL foods. Contrarily, a diet rich in low GI and low GL foods has been linked to better blood sugar regulation, effective weight management, and a decreased risk of chronic illnesses.

A healthy diet may be simple and pleasant to incorporate low GI and low GL items into. Legumes like lentils, chickpeas, and black beans, whole grains like quinoa, brown rice, and oats, as well as the majority of fruits and vegetables, are examples of low GI foods. The glycemic index of a meal can also be lowered by selecting high-fiber carbs, as they digest more gradually. The absorption of carbs can be slowed down and blood sugar rises prevented by consuming carbohydrates together with protein and healthy fats.

It is essential to remember that other parameters other than the glycemic index and glycemic load should be taken into account when choosing a diet. The nutritional content of foods, general dietary trends, and specific health objectives and requirements are further critical elements. A personalized nutrition plan can be developed by consulting a healthcare professional or registered dietitian to identify specific dietary requirements.

Finally, it should be noted that the glycemic index and glycemic load are crucial tools for comprehending how carbohydrates impact blood sugar levels. Managing blood sugar levels and lowering the risk of chronic illnesses can both benefit from using low GI and low GL items in a balanced diet. When choosing a diet, it's crucial to keep other aspects in mind. For more specific nutrition guidance, speak with a healthcare professional or registered dietitian.

How to interpret food labeling.

Making healthy meal selections may require you to read food labels. You may use it to better understand what you're putting in your body and choose a diet that suits your needs. Following are some pointers for reading food labels:

- Start by examining the serving size: The serving size should be the first item you examine on a food label. This will let you know how much food constitutes one serving and how many there are in the container. If you want to confirm that your nutrient consumption is accurate, make sure to compare the serving size to the quantity you consume.

- Analyze the calories: The total number of calories in each serving is the following consideration. This can help you estimate the amount of energy that a particular food item will provide. Pay attention to the calories from fat as well, as diets heavy in fat can cause weight gain and other health issues.

- Check the following part of the label for information on the food's macronutrient composition, which will often include information on the amount of fat, protein, and carbs. It's critical to remember that protein is a necessary part of a balanced diet and that not all fats are unhealthy. Make sure to thoroughly study labels to ascertain the kind and amount of macronutrients in your meal.

- Pay attention to the sugar level of the meals you consume. Sugar is often added to processed foods, and studies have shown that eating too much of it can lead to several health issues, including type 2 diabetes and obesity. Aim for items with little added sugar by carefully reading the sugar amount on food labels.

- Keep an eye out for fiber and other nutrients: Fiber is a crucial ingredient that may aid in digestion, control blood sugar levels, and encourage feelings of fullness. You should seek out meals that are high in fiber and other nutrients, such as vitamins and minerals.

- Look at the ingredient list: The list of components on food labels offers useful insight into the caliber of the item. Whenever possible, choose items with complete food components mentioned at the top and stay away from those that include preservatives, artificial sweeteners, and other additions.

- Analyze the brand: Not all food brands are created equally, and some could use ingredients of a higher caliber and adhere to more honest labeling procedures. Choose a brand after conducting research that emphasizes healthy, whole-food components.

- In general, reading food labels may be a crucial step in choosing nutritious foods. You may make educated choices about what you put in your body and give priority to a healthy, balanced diet by paying attention to serving sizes, calories, macronutrients, sugar content, fiber, ingredients, and brand.

Portion control

Controlling one's intake is essential for keeping a healthy diet. It entails controlling how much food you eat at each meal to avoid overeating or ingesting too many calories. Here is s some advice for exercising:

- Reduce portions by using smaller plates: Reducing portions is one of the simplest strategies to lose weight. This can aid in reducing your calorie intake while giving you the impression that you are eating a full plate of food.

- Measuring spoons, cups, and kitchen scales are helpful tools for helping you correctly measure your meal servings. This can be especially useful when it comes to items high in calories, such as nuts, cheese, and oils.

- Fill up on non-starchy veggies: Non-starchy vegetables, such as broccoli, carrots, and green beans, are low in calories and high in fiber, making them a great option for packing on the vegetables on your plate without going overboard with the calories.

- Eat mindfully: Mindful eating means paying attention to your food and the act of eating while being in the moment. This can aid improve your ability to recognize your body's signals of hunger and fullness, helping you avoid overeating.

- Avoid distractions when eating because doing so might result in mindless eating and overconsumption. Some examples of distractions while eating include watching TV or using your phone. To better focus on your meal, try to dine in a quiet setting free from interruptions.

- Pay attention to liquid calorie intake: Drinks like soda, juice, and alcohol may be rich in calories and cause overeating. Aim to drink water as your main beverage and keep an eye on the amount of these you consume.

- In the end, the secret to portion management is to pay attention to your body. Be mindful of your hunger and fullness signals, and stop eating when you are full rather than when your plate is finished.

- You may maintain a healthy weight, manage chronic conditions like diabetes and heart disease, and enhance your general health by using portion management techniques. You may effectively control your food intake and put a priority on a healthy, balanced diet by using smaller plates, weighing your food, stocking up on non-starchy veggies, engaging in mindful eating, staying focused while eating, being aware of liquid calories, and paying attention to your body.

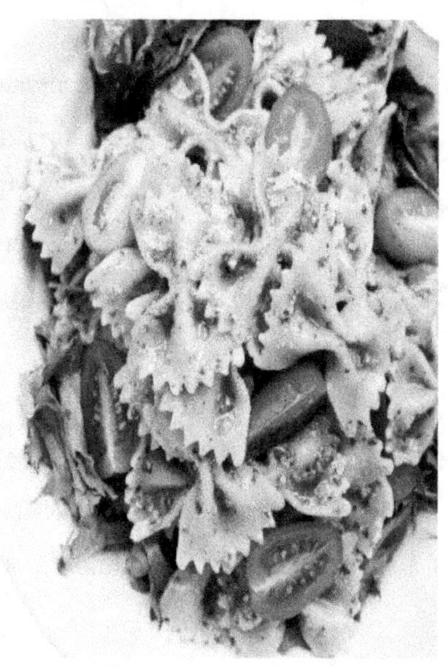

Chapter 4

Foods to limit or avoid if you have gestational diabetes

Food to avoid, e.g. foods with a high GI.

For those with gestational diabetes, maintaining adequate blood sugar levels is crucial. It's crucial to restrict or stay away from meals with a high glycemic index since they might raise blood sugar levels suddenly. The following foods should be avoided because of their high glycemic index:

- Refined carbs: Foods high in refined carbohydrates, such as white bread, white rice, and pasta, break down fast into glucose, causing a sharp rise in blood sugar levels.

- Sugary drinks: Sugar-rich drinks including soda, fruit juice, and energy drinks can raise blood sugar levels because of their high sugar content.

Candy, cake, cookies, and other sweets: Due to their high sugar content, sweets should either be avoided altogether or taken in moderation.

- Processed snacks: Chips, crackers, and other processed snacks should either be consumed in moderation or avoided due to their high levels of refined carbs.

- Morning cereals with added sugar: Since many morning cereals are heavy in sugar and processed carbs, they are not a good choice for those with gestational diabetes.

- Flavored yogurt should be avoided since it frequently contains a lot of added sugar. Choose plain Greek yogurt instead, and for sweetness, top with fresh fruit or a drizzle of honey.

- Fried foods: Fried meals like French fries, fried fish, fried chicken, and fried potatoes are frequently rich in calories, bad fats, and refined carbs, making them a bad choice for those with gestational diabetes.

- While it's crucial to minimize meals with a high glycemic index, it's also crucial to concentrate on including a range of healthful, nutrient-rich foods in your diet. These comprise:

- Vegetables that are not carbohydrates: Vegetables that are not carbohydrates, such as leafy greens, broccoli, and cauliflower, are low in calories and high in fiber and minerals.

- Whole grains: Foods high in fiber and minerals, including brown rice, quinoa, and whole-wheat bread, can help control blood sugar levels.

- Lean protein: Proteins with low-fat content, such as those found in chicken, fish, tofu, and beans, can make you feel full and satisfied while also supplying vital nutrients.

- Healthy fats: Foods high in healthy fats, such as avocado, nuts, seeds, and olive oil, can help control blood sugar levels while also supplying vital nutrients.

- Fruits with low sugar content: Berries, apples, and pears are examples of fresh fruits that are high in fiber and antioxidants and can help control blood sugar levels. The intake of fruits with high sugar content, such as grapes and bananas, should be kept to a minimum.

- A food's glycemic load, which takes into account both the glycemic index and the portion size, should also be considered. Even if they have a lower glycemic index, meals with a high glycemic load might result in a more pronounced rise in blood sugar levels than those with a lower glycemic load.

- Eat frequent meals and snacks throughout the day in addition to avoiding foods with a high glycemic index to maintain appropriate blood sugar levels. Additionally, this can lessen the likelihood of weight gain and binge eating, which both raise the risk of complications from gestational diabetes.

To create a nutritious food plan that suits your unique requirements and tastes while also controlling your gestational diabetes, talking to a qualified dietitian might be useful. Additionally, they may offer advice on portion management, how to read food labels, and how to choose nutritious foods while dining out.

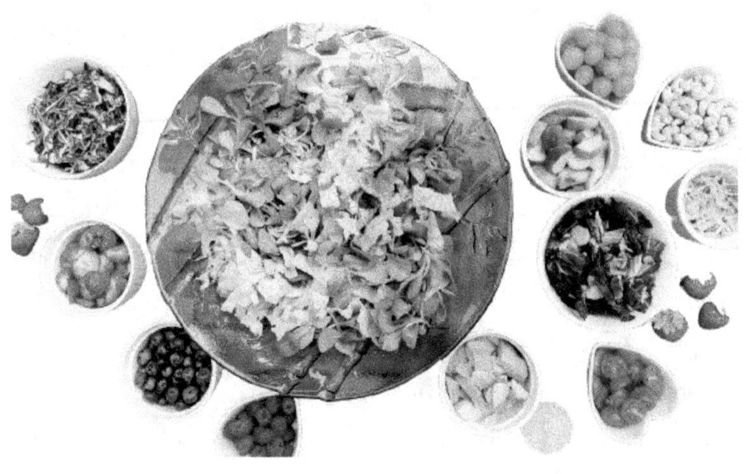

Integration of whole grains and complex carbs in the Gestational diet

Include whole grains and complex carbs in your diet if you have gestational diabetes to help keep your blood sugar levels in check. Because they are absorbed more slowly than refined carbs and are abundant in fiber, vitamins, and minerals, whole grains cause a steady rise in blood sugar levels. Additionally, significant providers of energy and minerals are complex carbohydrates, which include whole grains, veggies, and legumes.

To help you incorporate whole grains and complex carbs into your diet if you have gestational diabetes, here are some tips:

Pick whole grain bread instead of white bread: When choosing bread, go for whole grain. White bread has a higher glycemic index than whole grain bread, which has a higher fiber, vitamin, and mineral content.

Change from white to brown rice since it has more fiber and is a better source of complex carbs. It can also assist in controlling blood sugar levels, making it a better option for pregnant women who have gestational diabetes.

Add quinoa to your diet. Quinoa is a versatile grain that is high in protein and fiber, making it a fantastic choice for pregnant women. It may be substituted for rice or pasta in a variety of meals, as well as in salads and soups.

Include more legumes in your diet: Legumes, such as lentils, beans, and chickpeas, are low in glycemic index and high in fiber and protein. They may be included in casseroles, soups, stews, salads, and dressings for a nutritious and satisfying dinner.

Snack on whole grain crackers: For a healthy alternative to processed snacks like chips or crackers, select whole grain crackers or rice cakes.

When creating pasta recipes, select whole-grain pasta in place of conventional pasta. Pasta made from whole grains is lower in glycemic index and richer in fiber and minerals.

Try out various grains: To spice up your diet, try out various whole grains including quinoa, barley, bulgur, and farro.

You should be mindful of portion quantities while including healthy grains and complex carbs in your diet. Even healthful meals can raise blood sugar levels if they are taken in significant amounts. To identify the right types of whole grains and complex carbs to include in your diet, as well as the right portion amounts, speak with a qualified dietitian.

In addition to incorporating whole grains and complex carbohydrates, it's important to balance your meals with lean protein, healthy fats, and non-starchy vegetables. Eating a balanced meal with a combination of nutrients can help regulate blood sugar levels and prevent overeating.

Overall, including whole grains and complex carbohydrates in your gestational diabetes diet can help maintain healthy blood sugar levels, provide important nutrients, and contribute to overall health and wellness.

Inclusion of Fruits and vegetables in the gestational diet

Fruits and vegetables are an essential part of any healthy diet, and this is especially true for pregnant women with gestational diabetes. Fruits and vegetables are packed with vitamins, minerals, and fiber, which are all important for a healthy pregnancy. These foods can also help to regulate blood sugar levels and reduce the risk of complications during pregnancy. Here are some tips on how to include fruits and vegetables in your gestational diabetes diet.

Choose low glycemic index fruits and vegetables
When choosing fruits and vegetables for your gestational diabetes diet, it's important to consider the glycemic index (GI) of each food. The glycemic index is a measure of how fast food raises blood sugar levels. Foods with a high glycemic index can cause blood sugar levels to spike, which can be dangerous for women with gestational diabetes. On the other hand, foods with a low glycemic index can

help regulate blood sugar levels and reduce the risk of complications.

Some examples of low-GI fruits and vegetables include:

- Berries (strawberries, blueberries, raspberries)
- Apples
- Oranges
- Grapefruit
- Peaches
- Plums
- Cherries
- Kiwi fruit
- Tomatoes
- Spinach
- Broccoli
- Cauliflower
- Green beans
- Lettuce
- Include a variety of colors and types

It's important to include a variety of fruits and vegetables in your gestational diabetes diet to ensure you're getting all the necessary nutrients. Different colors of fruits and vegetables indicate different nutrients, so try to include a range of colors in your diet. For example, dark green vegetables like spinach and broccoli are rich in iron and calcium, while red and orange vegetables like carrots and sweet potatoes are high in vitamin A.

Incorporating fruits and vegetables into meals and snacks

There are many ways to incorporate fruits and vegetables into your gestational diabetes diet. You can add them to meals, snacks, or smoothies. For example, you can add spinach or kale to a morning smoothie, or snack on sliced apples with peanut butter. You can also add veggies to your omelet or wrap for a healthy breakfast or lunch option. For dinner, try roasting a variety of vegetables, such as broccoli, cauliflower, and carrots, for a delicious and nutritious side dish.

Be mindful of portion sizes

While fruits and vegetables are an important part of any healthy diet, it's still important to be mindful of portion sizes. Eating too much of any food can cause blood sugar levels to rise, so it's important to eat a balanced diet that includes a variety of foods in appropriate portions. A general guideline is to fill half of your plate with non-starchy vegetables, a quarter with protein, and a quarter with whole grains or starchy vegetables.

In conclusion, incorporating a variety of colorful and low glycemic index fruits and vegetables in appropriate portion sizes can help regulate blood sugar levels and reduce the risk of complications during pregnancy. Additionally, fruits and vegetables are packed with essential nutrients that are important for a healthy pregnancy. So, try to include these nutritious foods in your gestational diabetes diet to ensure a healthy pregnancy for you and your baby.

Inclusion of Lean proteins in the gestational diet

During pregnancy, getting enough protein is important for the growth and development of the baby, as well as for maintaining the mother's health. Lean protein sources can provide the necessary protein while keeping fat intake in check. Here are some tips on how to include lean protein sources in a gestational diet.

- Choose lean cuts of meat: When selecting meat, choose lean cuts such as chicken breast, turkey, pork tenderloin, and beef sirloin. These cuts contain less fat and more protein per serving compared to fattier cuts.

- Incorporate plant-based proteins: Plant-based proteins such as legumes, tofu, tempeh, and nuts are great sources of lean protein. They are also high in fiber and can help keep blood sugar levels stable. Try adding beans to soups and salads, or enjoy a tofu stir-fry.

Opt for seafood: Seafood is a great source of protein and healthy fats. Choose low-mercury options such as salmon, trout, sardines, and shrimp. These options are also rich in omega-3 fatty acids, which are essential for fetal brain development.

- Include dairy products: Dairy products such as milk, cheese, and yogurt are good sources of protein and calcium. Choose low-fat or fat-free options to keep fat intake in check.

- Add eggs to the diet: Eggs are a great source of high-quality protein and essential vitamins and minerals. Try making an omelet with vegetables or adding a hard-boiled egg to a salad.

Due to their high mercury level, several fish species, including swordfish, shark, and king mackerel, should be avoided during pregnancy. To lower their chance of contracting a foodborne disease, pregnant women should also stay away from eating raw or undercooked meat, poultry, shellfish, and eggs.

It's crucial to consider portion sizes in addition to selecting lean protein sources. A portion of protein generally weighs 3 to 4 ounces or the equivalent of a deck of cards. Depending on their weight and amount of exercise, pregnant women need between 75 and 100 grams of protein each day.

Lean protein sources may assist guarantee that both the mother and the unborn child are receiving the nutrients they need for good health by including them in a gestational diet. For individualized advice on protein consumption during pregnancy, speak with a medical professional or a qualified dietitian.

How to include lean, healthy fats into your diet during pregnancy.

For the mother's health as well as the growth of the baby's brain and nervous system, including healthy fats in a gestational diet is crucial. But it's crucial to choose healthy sources of fat and use them sparingly. Here are some suggestions for adding lean, healthy fats to your diet during pregnancy.

- Pick plant-based oils: These oils are excellent sources of healthy fats and include coconut oil, avocado oil, and olive oil. Use them to make salad dressings or as a culinary ingredient.

- Include fatty fish: Omega-3 fatty acids, which are vital for embryonic brain and nervous system development, are abundant in fatty fish like salmon, sardines, and trout. Two portions of fatty fish should be consumed per week.

- Include nuts and seeds: Nuts and seeds are excellent sources of fiber, protein, and healthy fats. Include a handful of almonds or walnuts as a snack, or top oatmeal or yogurt with chia seeds or flaxseeds.

- Select lean cuts of meat since they contain beneficial fats in moderation, such as chicken breast, turkey, and beef sirloin. With a little oil, try grilling or roasting these chops.

- Include avocado in your meals since it is an excellent source of fiber, healthy fats, and other vital elements. Make guacamole as a nutritious snack or serve slices of avocado on sandwiches or in salads.

- Although healthy fats are necessary, it's vital to remember that they should still be ingested in proportion. Ideally, pregnant women should take 20 to 35 percent of their daily calories as fat, with the bulk of those calories coming from nutritious foods including nuts, seeds, fatty fish, almonds, and plant-based oils.

- Additionally, it's critical to stay away from harmful forms of fat including trans and saturated fats. The chance of developing gestational diabetes, high blood pressure, and other health problems might rise as a result of these lipids. Fried meals, fatty meats, and processed snacks are examples of sources of harmful fats.

- A qualified dietitian or healthcare professional may provide specific suggestions for adding healthy fats to a prenatal diet. Per each person's requirements and preferences, they may also provide advice on suitable portion sizes and total calorie consumption.

In conclusion, eating lean, healthy fats in a prenatal diet may help the mother and growing baby get the nutrients they need. Pregnant women may encourage the best health and development for both themselves and their unborn children by selecting healthy sources of fat and eating them in moderation.

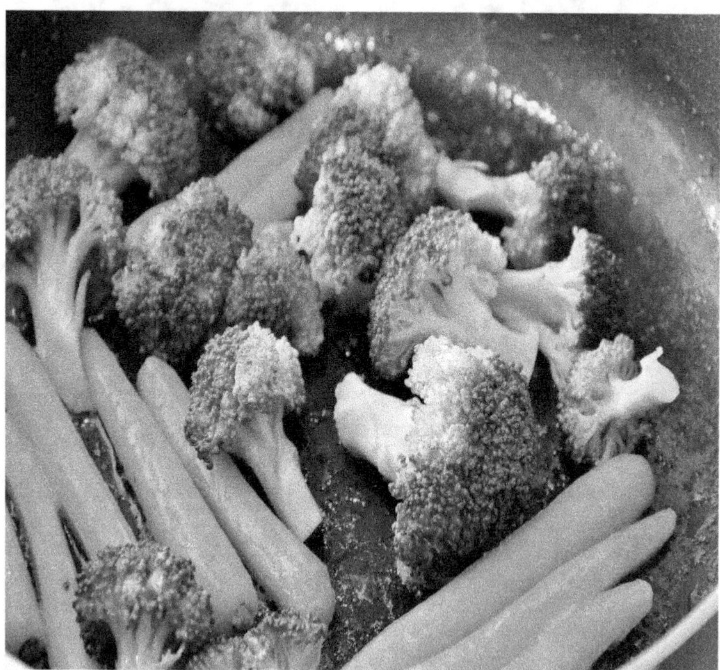

Chapter 5

Meal plans during the Gestation

Breakfast for Gestational Diabetes

Here is a breakfast meal suitable for those with gestational diabetes from Lily Nichols' "Gestational Diabetes Cookbook: 101 Delicious, Low-Carb Recipes for the Healthiest Pregnancy":

Vegetable and Egg Scramble

Ingredients:

1. two huge eggs

2. Chopped red bell pepper, 1/4 cup

3. 1 cup of finely chopped zucchini

4. 14 cups finely minced onion

5. 1-tablespoon olive oil

6. dried basil, 1/4 teaspoon

7. pepper and salt as desired

Instructions:

- In a small dish, whisk the eggs; put aside.
- In a nonstick skillet over medium heat, warm the olive oil.
- The chopped veggies should be added and sautéed for 3 to 4 minutes, or until tender.
- Stirring carefully, add the whisked eggs to the pan with the veggies.
- Add the dried basil and taste-test adding salt and pepper.
- For approximately 3 to 4 minutes, cook the eggs, stirring regularly, until they are set and well-cooked.
- Enjoy your breakfast that is suitable for gestational diabetes while it is hot!

Smoothie with yogurt and berries

Ingredients:

1. 1 cup of unflavored Greek yogurt
2. 1/2 cup of berries (such as strawberries, blueberries, and raspberries)
3. 2 tablespoons chopped walnuts
4. (Optional) 1 teaspoon of honey

Instructions:

- The berries should be rinsed and dried with paper towels.
- Yogurt, berries, and chopped walnuts should be arranged in layers in a glass or dish.
- If you want, drizzle with honey.
- Right away serve.
- For ladies with gestational diabetes, this breakfast recipe's low-carb and high-protein content makes it a fantastic choice. Enjoy!

Reduced-Carb Veggie Frittata

Ingredients:

1. Large eggs, four
2. 1/2 cup chopped red pepper 1/2 cup chopped onion
3. 14 finely chopped zucchini
4. 1 tablespoon of olive oil
5. 1/four teaspoon dried oregano
6. As desired, add salt and pepper.

Instructions:

- The oven should be heated to 375°F (190°C).
- Make sure the eggs are well beaten in a mixing basin.
- A nonstick skillet with medium heat is used to warm the olive oil.
- After adding, sauté the veggies for 3–4 minutes, or until they soften.
- The eggs should be whisked and then poured over the skillet's veggies.
- Over the top, sprinkle dry oregano.
- According to taste, add salt and pepper.
- Bake for 10 to 12 minutes, or until the eggs are set, in the preheated oven with the skillet inside.
- Take out it of the oven, and then give the food some time to cool.
- Serve wedge-style after cutting.

- For pregnant women with gestational diabetes, this tasty and nutritious low-carb vegetable frittata is a great alternative. Enjoy!

Almond and berry oatmeal

Ingredients:

1. Rolling oats, half a cup
2. A cup of water
3. One-fourth cup of mixed nuts, such as almonds, pecans, and walnuts
4. 14 berries (such as strawberries, blueberries, and raspberries)
5. (Optional) 1 tablespoon of honey

Instructions:

- Boiling water is accomplished in a pan.
- Change the heat to medium after adding the rolled oats.
- The oats will thicken after cooking for 5-7 minutes with sporadic stirring.

- The berries should be rinsed and dried with paper towels.
- cut the nuts roughly.
- As you mix the oats, add the chopped nuts and berries.
- If you want, drizzle with honey.
- Offer hot.

Poached eggs with avocado toast

Ingredients:

1. two pieces of whole grain bread
2. one ripe avocado
3. 2 big eggs
4. 1 tablespoon white vinegar
5. To taste with salt and pepper

Instructions:

- Toasted bread should be done to your preference.
- After halving the avocado, scrape the flesh into a small mixing dish and remove the pit.
- Use a fork to thoroughly mash the avocado.
- Pepper and salt should be added for seasoning.
- 2 inches of water should be simmering in a small pot.
- Water is added along with white vinegar.
- The eggs should be cracked into several ramekins or bowls.

- In the simmering water, stir a soft whirlpool with a spoon.

- One egg should be slowly added to the whirlpool's center.

- When the white of the egg is set but the yolk is still runny, let it cook for 3–4 minutes.

- Carefully take the poached egg from the water with a slotted spoon, then set it on some paper towels to absorb any remaining water.

- With the second egg, repeat steps 9 through 11.

- Toast pieces are covered with mashed avocado.

- Poached eggs are placed on top of each piece.

- Add more pepper and salt to your taste.

- Serve immediately.

- For pregnant women with gestational diabetes, this avocado toast with poached eggs is a delicious and wholesome choice. Enjoy!

Vegetable smoothie

Ingredients:

1. Unsweetened almond milk in 1/2 cup

2. 50 g of baby spinach

3. 50% of a cup of frozen mixed berries

4. 14 avocado

5. a tablespoon of ground flaxseed

6. (Optional) Half a scoop of vanilla protein powder

Instructions:

- Baby spinach, frozen mixed berries, avocado, ground flaxseed, and protein powder (if used) may all be added to a blender along with almond milk.
- Blend until well combined and creamy.
- Add additional almond milk if the smoothie is too thick until you have the ideal consistency.
- In a glass, pour the smoothie.
- Serve immediately.
- For ladies with gestational diabetes, this green smoothie is a delightful and wholesome breakfast choice. It has a low carbohydrate content and is strong in protein, healthy fats, and fiber. Enjoy!

Pancakes with Greek Yogurt

Ingredients:

1. Greek yogurt, plain, one cup

2. 1/2 cup of mixed berries, including strawberries, blueberries, and raspberries

3. Almonds, pecans, and walnuts, in the amount of 1/4 cup, chopped

4. 1 teaspoon of optional honey

Instructions:

- Wash the berries and pat them dry.
- the nuts into rough pieces.
- Greek yogurt and honey (if used) should be combined in a small mixing dish.
- In a glass or dish, arrange the yogurt, chopped almonds, and mixed berries.
- Till all components are used, keep adding layers.
- Serve immediately.
- For pregnant women with gestational diabetes, this Greek yogurt parfait is a delightful and healthful breakfast alternative. It has a low carbohydrate content and is strong in fiber, healthy fats, and protein. Enjoy!

Veggie Frittata

Ingredients:

1. 6 big eggs

2. 1/2 cup of finely chopped veggies, such as spinach, bell pepper, and onion

3. Parmesan cheese, grated, two tablespoons

4. Olive oil, one tablespoon

5. To taste with salt and pepper

Instructions:

- Achieve a 375°F (190°C) oven temperature.

- The eggs should be well mixed in a mixing basin.

- The eggs should also have Parmesan cheese added.

- Add pepper and salt to taste when seasoning.

- Heat the olive oil o medium-high heat in an oven-safe skillet.

- To the skillet, add the egg and veggie combination.

- The edges should start to firm after 3–4 minutes of cooking.

- Bake the frittata for 10 to 12 minutes, or until it is set in the center and the top is browned brown, in the preheated oven.

- After taking the skillet out of the oven, give it some time to cool.

- Slide the frittata onto a chopping board using a spatula.

- Slices are then served.

- Women with gestational diabetes may have a filling and healthy breakfast with this veggie frittata. It has a low carbohydrate content and is strong in fiber and protein. Enjoy!

Chapter 6

Meal plans during the Gestation

Lunch for Gestational Diabetes

Chickpea Salad from the Middle East

Ingredients:

1. chickpeas from one can, washed and drained
2. 1/4 cup pitted and sliced kalamata olives, 1/2 diced cucumber, 1/2 diced red onion, 1/2 diced bell pepper, 1/2 cup halved cherry tomatoes
3. Crumbled feta cheese, 2 tablespoons
4. 2 tablespoons of fresh parsley, chopped
5. Fresh mint, chopped, 1 tablespoon
6. Olive oil, one tablespoon

7. 2 tablespoons lemon juice

8. To taste with salt and pepper

Instructions:

- Chickpeas, cucumber, red onion, bell pepper, cherry tomatoes, and kalamata olives should all be combined in a large mixing dish.

- The mixing dish should now include the feta cheese crumbles, chopped parsley, and chopped mint.

- Olive oil, lemon juice, salt, and pepper should all be combined in a separate, small mixing dish.

- Toss the chickpea salad with the dressing until everything is evenly covered.

- You may either serve the salad right now or chill it until you're ready to.

- For pregnant women with gestational diabetes, this Mediterranean chickpea salad is a tasty and healthy lunch alternative. It is low in carbs and abundant in healthy fats, fiber, and protein. Enjoy!

- Certainly, the following lunch meal from Lily Nichols' "Gestational Diabetes Cookbook" is acceptable for gestational diabetes:

Avocado and Salmon Salad

Ingredients:

1. 4 ounces of fish that have been a grill
2. 2 cups baby kale
3. sliced half an avocado
4. halved 1/4 cup cherry tomatoes
5. Cucumber, diced, 14 cup
6. Chopped fresh dill, 1 tablespoon
7. Olive oil, one tablespoon
8. 2 tablespoons lemon juice
9. To taste with salt and pepper

Instructions:

- In a big salad dish, add the baby spinach.
- On top of the spinach, scatter the cherry tomatoes, chopped cucumber, and avocado slices.
- The grilled salmon should be flaked and added to the salad.
- Olive oil, lemon juice, salt, and pepper should all be combined in a small mixing dish.
- When the salad is well covered, pour the dressing over it and toss.
- Add freshly chopped dill on top of the salad.
- You may either serve the salad right now or chill it until you're ready to.

- For ladies with gestational diabetes, this salmon and avocado salad is a delightful and healthful lunch alternative. It has a low carbohydrate content and is strong in fiber, healthy fats, and protein. Enjoy!

Stir-fried vegetables with chicken

Ingredients:

1. 4 oz. sliced boneless, skinless chicken breast
2. a half-cup of broccoli florets
3. a half-cup of sliced bell peppers
4. Sliced onion, 1/4 cup
5. Carrots, cut, 14 cup
6. Olive oil, one tablespoon
7. Reduced-sodium soy sauce, 1 tablespoon
8. 1/9 cup rice vinegar
9. 1 minced clove of garlic
10. Grated fresh ginger, half a teaspoon

Instructions:

- The olive oil should be heated over medium-high in a large skillet or wok.
- Sliced chicken should be added to the pan and stir-fried for 5-7 minutes, or until cooked through.

- The cooked chicken should be taken out of the pan and put aside.
- To the pan, add the bell pepper, onion, bell peppers, and carrot slices in slices.
- To make the veggies tender, stir-fry them for 5-7 minutes.
- Stir-fry the minced garlic and grated ginger for one to two minutes in the skillet.
- Reintroduce the cooked chicken to the skillet.
- Rice vinegar and low-sodium soy sauce should be combined in a small mixing dish.
- The chicken and veggies in the pan will be covered with the soy sauce mixture.
- Stir-fry everything for 1-2 minutes, or until everything is completely covered with sauce.
- Over a bed of brown rice or quinoa, serve the stir-fry right away.
- For pregnant women with gestational diabetes, this stir-fry of chicken and vegetables is a fast and simple lunch alternative. It has a low carbohydrate content and is strong in fiber and protein. Enjoy!
-

Wraps with tuna salad

Ingredients:

1. 1 drained can (5 oz) of tuna

2. chopped celery, 2 tablespoons

3. 2 tbsp. red onion, diced

4. 1-tablespoon mayonnaise

5. mustard, Dijon, 1 teaspoon

6. To taste with salt and pepper

7. four big lettuce leaves

Instructions:

- Combine the drained tuna, chopped celery, diced red onion, mayonnaise, Dijon mustard, salt, and pepper in a small mixing dish.
- Combine all of the ingredients well.
- On each of the four big lettuce leaves, distribute the tuna salad equally.
- To make wraps, roll up the lettuce leaves.
- The tuna salad lettuce wraps may be served right away or stored in the refrigerator until needed.
- Women with gestational diabetes might enjoy this tuna salad lettuce wraps as a nutritious and low-carb lunch choice. They have fewer carbs and a lot of protein and good fats. Enjoy!

Asparagus and Salmon Salad

Ingredients:

1. Salmon fillet, 4 ounces
2. 50 g of asparagus spears
3. a half-cup of mixed greens
4. Olive oil, one tablespoon
5. a tablespoon of balsamic vinegar
6. mustard, Dijon, 1 teaspoon
7. To taste with salt and pepper

Instructions:

- The Fahrenheit should be set at 400 degrees for the oven.
- The salmon fillet should be put on a baking pan covered with parchment paper.
- Olive oil and salt and pepper to taste should be drizzled over the fish.
- For 12 to 15 minutes, or until thoroughly done, roast the fish in the oven.
- Olive oil, balsamic vinegar, Dijon mustard, salt, and pepper should all be combined in a small mixing dish.
- Asparagus spears should be steamed till tender-crisp.
- The mixed greens and cooked asparagus should be combined in a large mixing dish.
- Combine the mixed greens and asparagus with the balsamic vinaigrette by drizzling it over everything.

- The cooked salmon should be flaked into bite-sized pieces.

- Separate the asparagus and mixed greens between the two dishes.

- Flaked salmon should be placed on each dish.

- Serve the salad of salmon and asparagus right away.

- For ladies with gestational diabetes, this salmon and asparagus salad is a filling and delicious lunch alternative. It has a low carbohydrate content and is strong in fiber, healthy fats, and protein. Enjoy!

The turkey and vegetable wrap

Ingredients:

1. 1 wrap with whole grain
2. Turkey breast cut into 2 oz.
3. Sliced 1/4 avocado
4. Sliced cucumber in 1/4 cup
5. Red bell peppers cut into 1/4 cup
6. a quarter cup of young spinach leaves
7. hummus, one tablespoon

Instructions:

- On a plate or cutting board, place the tortilla wrap flat.

- Over the whole tortilla wrap, spread a thin coating of hummus.
- The hummus is topped with thinly sliced turkey, avocado, cucumber, red bell pepper, and baby spinach leaves.
- The sides should be tucked in as you securely roll the tortilla wrap.
- Serve right away after cutting the wrap in half diagonally.
- For pregnant women with gestational diabetes, this turkey and vegetable wrap is a tasty and healthful lunch alternative. Low in carbs and abundant in fiber, protein, good fats, and vitamins. Enjoy!

Veggie and Chicken Kebabs on the Grill

Ingredients:

1. Skinless, boneless chicken breast, 4 ounces
2. big slices of a 1/4 red onion
3. big slices of a half-red bell pepper
4. big slices of half of a yellow bell pepper
5. thick circles of half a zucchini
6. Olive oil, one tablespoon
7. a tablespoon of balsamic vinegar
8. mustard, Dijon, 1 teaspoon
9. To taste with salt and pepper

Instructions:

- Warm up the grill to a medium-high setting.
- Make bite-sized pieces out of the chicken breast.
- On skewers, arrange the chicken, red onion, red bell pepper, yellow bell pepper, and zucchini.
- Olive oil, balsamic vinegar, Dijon mustard, salt, and pepper should all be combined in a small mixing dish.
- The chicken and vegetables on the skewers should be covered with balsamic vinaigrette.
- The kebabs should be grilled for 10 to 12 minutes, rotating once, or until the chicken is well-cooked and the vegetables are soft.
- Serve the kebabs right away after removing them from the grill.
- Women with gestational diabetes may enjoy these savory and nutritious grilled chicken and vegetable kebabs for lunch. They have a low carbohydrate content and a high protein, fiber, vitamin, and mineral content. Enjoy!

Wraps with tuna salad

Ingredients:

1. 2 cans of drained tuna in water
2. chopped celery, 1/4 cup

3. Red onion, chopped, in 1/4 cup

4. 1/4 cup mayonnaise and 1 tablespoon freshly chopped dill

5. To taste with salt and pepper

6. four big lettuce leaves

Instructions:

- Combine the drained tuna, mayonnaise, salt, pepper, diced celery, diced red onion, and chopped dill in a medium mixing dish.
- Mix well until all components are distributed equally.
- A huge lettuce leaf should be placed on a dish or cutting board.
- Onto the lettuce leaf, heap a large quantity of the tuna salad.
- The tuna salad should be wrapped in lettuce, with the edges tucked in as you roll.
- Use the remaining lettuce leaves and tuna salad in the same manner.
- The tuna salad lettuce wraps should be served right away.
- Women with gestational diabetes might enjoy this tuna salad lettuce wraps as a filling lunch alternative. They include fewer carbs and a lot of protein, good fats, vitamins, and minerals. Enjoy!

Chapter 7

Meal plans during the Gestation

Dinner for Gestational Diabetes

Roasted vegetables and salmon

Ingredients:

1. Salmon fillet, wild-caught, 4 oz.
2. Red bell pepper cut into strips and a medium-sized sweet potato that has been peeled and cubed
3. Sliced into strips, half a yellow bell pepper
4. Round slices of half a zucchini
5. Olive oil, one tablespoon
6. Dry thyme, 1 teaspoon
7. To taste with salt and pepper

Instructions:

- The Fahrenheit should be set at 400 decors the oven.
- Put parchment paper on a baking pan to line it.
- On the baking sheet, spread out the cubed sweet potato, thinly sliced bell peppers, and thinly sliced zucchini.
- Olive oil, salt, and pepper, along with dried thyme, should be drizzled over the veggies.
- Toss the veggies to distribute the oil and spices evenly.
- The veggies should be baked for 20 to 25 minutes, or until they are soft and beginning to caramelize.
- Over medium heat, preheat a nonstick skillet.
- Pepper and salt should be added to the salmon fillet.
- Cook the salmon fillet for 4-5 minutes with the skin side down in the pan.
- Once cooked through, flip the salmon fillet over and cook for an additional 2 to 3 minutes.
- Roasted veggies should be served with the fish.
- For ladies with gestational diabetes, this salmon dish with roasted veggies is a wholesome and filling supper alternative. It has a low carbohydrate content while being abundant in fiber, vitamins, minerals, and omega-3 fatty acids. Enjoy!

Stir-fried vegetables with chicken

Ingredients:

1. 4 ounces of thinly sliced, skinless, and boneless chicken breast
2. thin pieces of half of a red bell pepper
3. thin pieces of half of a yellow bell pepper
4. a half-cup of broccoli florets
5. a half-cup of sliced mushrooms
6. 1-tablespoon coconut oil
7. minced one garlic clove
8. 1 teaspoon freshly grated ginger
9. 1-tablespoon tamari sauce
10. To taste with salt and pepper

Instructions:

- Over medium-high heat, preheat a nonstick skillet.
- After adding, let the coconut oil melt.
- The chicken should be cooked through and browned when you add the sliced chicken breast to the pan and stir-fry for 2–3 minutes.
- For a further 2-3 minutes, or until the veggies are tender-crisp, add the sliced bell peppers, broccoli florets, and mushrooms to the skillet.

- Stir together the pan contents after adding the minced garlic, grated ginger, tamari sauce, salt, and pepper.
- Once the sauce has thickened and covered the chicken and veggies, cook for another minute or two.
- Serve the stir-fried chicken and vegetables right away.
- For pregnant women with gestational diabetes, this dish of chicken and vegetables makes a delightful and nutritious lunch alternative. Low in carbs and abundant in protein, fiber, vitamins, and minerals. Enjoy!

Burger made with grilled turkey and salad

Ingredients:

1. Turkey meat, 4 ounces
2. coarsely sliced 1/4 of a tiny red onion
3. Garlic powder, 1/4 teaspoon
4. Ground cumin, 1/4 teaspoon
5. To taste with salt and pepper
6. 1 serving of mixed salad greens
7. slice of a medium cucumber, 1/4
8. Sliced 1/4 medium tomato, 1 tablespoon extra-virgin olive oil
9. 2 tablespoons of apple cider vinegar
10. 1/8 teaspoon of Dijon mustard
11. To taste with salt and pepper

Instructions:

- Over medium-high heat, preheat a nonstick skillet.
- After adding, let the coconut oil melt.
- The chicken should be cooked through and browned when you add the sliced chicken breast to the pan and stir-fry for 2–3 minutes.
- For a further 2-3 minutes, or until the veggies are tender-crisp, add the sliced bell peppers, broccoli florets, and mushrooms to the skillet.
- Stir together the pan contents after adding the minced garlic, grated ginger, tamari sauce, salt, and pepper.
- Once the sauce has thickened and covered the chicken and veggies, cook for another minute or two.
- Serve the stir-fried chicken and vegetables right away.
- For pregnant women with gestational diabetes, this dish f chicken and vegetables makes a delightful and nutritious lunch alternative. Low in carbs and abundant in protein, fiber, vitamins, and minerals. Enjoy!

Burger made with grilled turkey and salad

Ingredients:

1. Turkey meat, 4 ounces
2. coarsely sliced 1/4 of a tiny red onion
3. Garlic powder, 1/4 teaspoon
4. Ground cumin, 1/4 teaspoon
5. To taste with salt and pepper
6. 1 serving of mixed salad greens
7. slice of a medium cucumber, 1/4
8. Sliced 1/4 medium tomato, 1 tablespoon extra-virgin olive oil
9. 2 tablespoons of apple cider vinegar
10. 1/8 teaspoon of Dijon mustard
11. To taste with salt and pepper

Instructions:

- Over med-high heat, preheat a grill or grill pan.
- Combine the ground turkey with the minced red onion, cumin, garlic powder, salt, and pepper in a mixing bowl.
- Make a patty by thoroughly combining.
- The turkey patty should be cooked through, about 4-5 minutes on each side.

- Mix the mixed greens, cucumber, and tomato slices in a bowl to make the salad in the meanwhile.
- Olive oil, apple cider vinegar, Dijon mustard, salt, and pepper should all be combined in a small mixing dish.
- Over the salad, drizzle the dressing and toss to combine.
- The mixed salad should be served with the grilled turkey burger.
- For pregnant women with gestational diabetes, this dish for grilled turkey burgers with salad offers a filling and delicious lunch choice. Low in carbs and abundant in protein, fiber, vitamins, and minerals. Enjoy!

Avocado and Chicken Salad

Ingredients:

1. two cups of mixed salad greens
2. Cooked 4 oz. chicken breast, chopped 1/2 medium avocado, 1/4 small red onion, 1/4 cup cherry tomatoes, and 1 tablespoon extra-virgin olive oil
3. a tablespoon of balsamic vinegar
4. 1/4 teaspoon of Dijon mustard
5. To taste with salt and pepper

Instructions:

- Sliced chicken breast, diced avocado, sliced red onion, and split cherry tomatoes should all be combined with the mixed salad greens in a large mixing basin.

- Olive oil, balsamic vinegar, Dijon mustard, salt, and pepper should all be combined in a small mixing dish.

- Over the salad, drizzle the dressing and toss to combine.

- Serve immediately.

- Given that it is strong in protein, healthy fats, fiber, and vital vitamins and minerals while being low in carbs, this chicken and avocado salad is a fantastic lunch choice for pregnant women with gestational diabetes. Additionally, it is tasty and simple to make. Enjoy!

Vegetable and Lentil Soup

Ingredients:

1. Olive oil, one tablespoon
2. 1 medium carrot, diced, along with 1/2 small onion, 2 minced garlic cloves, and
3. 1 cup finely chopped celery
4. 0.5 cup finely sliced zucchini
5. a half-cup of chopped green beans
6. washed and drained 1/2 cup of dry lentils
7. 4 cups of vegetable or chicken broth low in salt
8. 0.5 teaspoon dried oregano

9. Dry thyme, half a teaspoon

10. To taste with salt and pepper

Instructions:

- Over medium heat, warm the olive oil in a big saucepan.

- Garlic and onion, both chopped, should be added and sautéed until the onion is transparent.

- For 5-7 minutes, while stirring periodically, add the chopped carrot, celery, zucchini, and green beans.

- Stir thoroughly after adding the salt, pepper, dried thyme, dried oregano, dry lentils, and chicken or vegetable broth.

- The soup should be brought to a boil, then simmer for 30 to 40 minutes, depending on how soft you want your lentils and veggies.

- Serve the food hot after seasoning to taste.

- For pregnant women with gestational diabetes, this lentil and vegetable soup is a filling and healthful lunch alternative. It has less sugar and fat and is high in fiber, protein, vitamins, and minerals. Additionally, it's simple to make and may be kept for later use in the freezer or refrigerator. Enjoy!

Salad with avocado and tuna

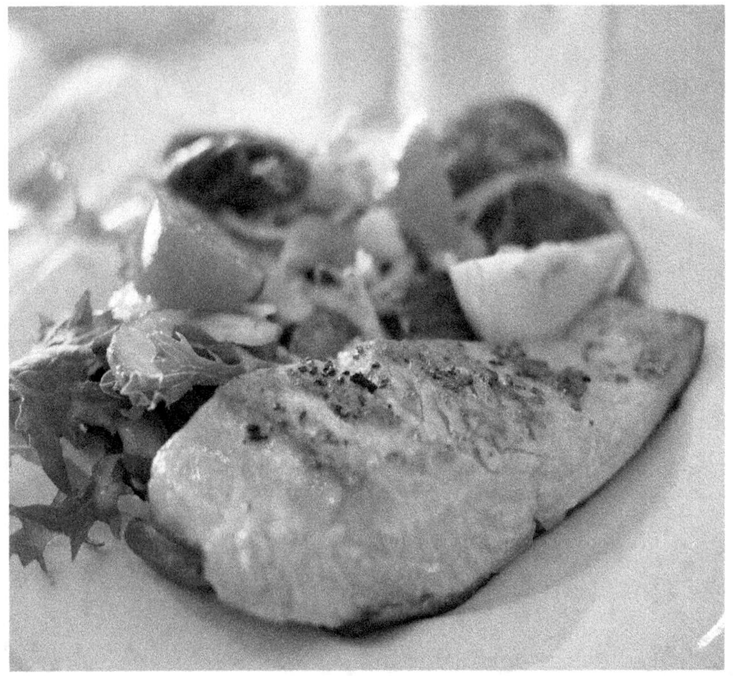

Ingredients:

1. 1 ripe avocado, peeled, and chopped, two water-packed 5 oz. cans of tuna, and

2. diced half a red onion

3. chopped red bell pepper, half

4. Fresh parsley, 1/4 cup, chopped

5. A quarter cup of chopped fresh cilantro

6. a tablespoon of fresh lime juice

7. Olive oil, two tablespoons

8. To taste with salt and pepper

Instructions:

- Combine the drained tuna with the diced avocado, red onion, diced bell pepper, chopped fresh parsley, and chopped fresh cilantro in a medium bowl.

- To create the dressing, combine the olive oil, salt, and pepper in a small bowl with the fresh lime juice.

- Then, douse the tuna and avocado combination with the dressing and gently toss to incorporate.

- You can either serve the tuna and avocado salad right away or chill it in the fridge for 30 to 60 minutes.

- Women with gestational diabetes might enjoy this tuna and avocado salad as a filling lunch alternative. It is low in carbs and salt and high in protein, good fats, vitamins, and minerals. Additionally, it's simple to modify by using or omitting additional veggies or herbs following your taste preferences. Enjoy!

Stir-fried vegetables with chicken

Ingredients:

1. 1 tablespoon of coconut or olive oil
2. 2 cups chopped veggies (including broccoli, snow peas, carrots, and mushrooms), 2 cloves minced garlic, 1 bell pepper, and 1 cup sliced onion
3. Sliced chicken breast from 1
4. To taste with salt and pepper
5. a half-cup of low-sodium soy sauce
6. Honey, one tablespoon
7. 1 tablespoon grated ginger
8. 1 teaspoon sesame oil

Instructions:

- In a large skillet or wok set over medium-high heat, warm the coconut oil or olive oil.
- Add the minced garlic and onion slices, and sauté for one to two minutes until aromatic.
- Stir-fry the veggies in the pan with the bell pepper slices for 2 to 3 minutes, or until they start to soften.
- Salt and pepper the chicken breast slices before adding them to the pan. Cook through after 5-7 minutes of stirring.

- To create the sauce, combine the honey, ginger, sesame oil, and low-sodium soy sauce in a small bowl.

- Stirring is necessary after adding the sauce to the stir-fried chicken and vegetables.

- With brown rice or quinoa, if preferred, serve the stir-fry hot.

- This protein-, fiber-, and a healthy fat-rich stir-fry of chicken and vegetables has a minimal salt and carbohydrate content. It's a wonderful choice for lunch that is not only nutritious but also savory and filling.

Wraps with tuna salad

Ingredients:

1. 1 drained can (5 oz) of tuna
2. chopped celery, 1/4 cup
3. Red onion, chopped, in 1/4 cup
4. Mayo, two tablespoons
5. 1 tsp. Dillon mustard
6. To taste with salt and pepper
7. four big lettuce leaves

Instructions:

- Tuna, celery, red onion, mayonnaise, Dijon mustard, salt, and pepper should all be combined in a small bowl.

- A lettuce leaf should be placed on a plate, and the middle of the leaf should be topped with 1/4 of the tuna salad mixture.

- To create a wrap, fold the lettuce leaf over the tuna salad mixture.

- Repetition is required with the rest of the lettuce leaves and tuna salad mixture.

- If preferred, serve cherry tomatoes or cucumber slices on the side with the tuna salad lettuce wraps.

- This recipe for tuna salad lettuce wraps is strong in protein and good fats, low in carbs, and contains fiber and omega-3 fatty acids, two necessary elements. It's a fast and simple lunch option that can be made in advance and consumed at home or work.

Chicken Salad in the Middle East

Ingredients:

1. cooked, diced one cup of chicken breast
2. 200 ml of mixed greens
3. Cucumber, diced, 14 cup
4. Cherry tomatoes, diced, 14 cup

5. Feta cheese crumbles, 1/4 cup

6. Fresh parsley, chopped, 1 tablespoon

7. Chopped fresh basil, one tablespoon

8. Olive oil, extra virgin, two tablespoons

9. a tablespoon of balsamic vinegar

10. To taste with salt and pepper

Instructions:

- Cooked chicken, mixed greens, cucumber, cherry tomatoes, feta cheese, parsley, and basil should all be combined in a big dish.

- Olive oil, balsamic vinegar, salt, and pepper should all be combined in a small basin.

- The salad should be tossed after the dressing has been added.

- If preferred, top with more fresh herbs before serving right away.

- A balanced lunch with plenty of protein, fiber, and good fats is this Mediterranean chicken salad. It's also low in carbs, which makes it a fantastic option for pregnant women who are diabetic. You may alter the salad by including or excluding certain veggies or herbs, and it's a fantastic way to sample a range of tastes and textures.

Section 8

Gestational Diabetes and Exercise

An essential part of controlling gestational diabetes is regularly checking blood sugar levels. To make sure their blood sugar levels remain within a reasonable range, pregnant women with gestational diabetes should periodically check their blood sugar levels. When monitoring blood sugar levels throughout pregnancy, it's important to have the following considerations in mind.

Maintain a schedule: A precise regimen for checking blood sugar levels will probably be advised by your doctor or certified dietician. Testing may be done in this manner one hour before meals, one hour after meals, and before bed. To guarantee accurate findings, it's crucial to adhere to this plan continuously.

Use a glucose meter to check your blood sugar levels. A glucose meter is a little instrument that does just that. On how to appropriately use a glucose meter, you may get advice from your doctor or a trained dietician.

Observe trends and note any problems by keeping a record of your blood sugar levels. Make careful to note the day and time of each test, as well as any other pertinent details like your diet and if you exercised.

Follow a meal plan: Maintaining blood sugar levels within a healthy range may be accomplished by adhering to a healthy diet plan. A specific meal plan that suits your requirements might be recommended by a trained dietician or your healthcare practitioner.

Take medicine as directed: Medications may sometimes be required to help regulate blood sugar levels. Make careful to follow the directions on any prescription drugs that your doctor gives you.

Speak with your healthcare professional or a certified dietitian if you observe any unexpected blood sugar readings or have concerns about your blood sugar levels. They may advise you on any changes that need to be made to your diet or medicines.

Ketones are created as the body breaks down fat for energy and may be dangerous if they accumulate in the blood. Especially if their blood sugar levels are continuously high, pregnant women with gestational diabetes should periodically check their ketone levels.

To sum up, keeping an eye on blood sugar levels is an essential part of controlling gestational diabetes. Women who have gestational diabetes during pregnancy may maintain appropriate blood sugar levels by adhering to a routine, using a glucose meter, keeping a diary, following a diet plan, taking prescribed medication, and seeking medical guidance as necessary. This may lower the risk of issues related to gestational diabetes and support the mother's and growing baby's best health.

How to regulate blood sugar levels through food and exercise

A kind of diabetes called gestational diabetes may develop during pregnancy. To guarantee the best possible health for both the mother and the unborn child, blood sugar levels during pregnancy must be kept under control. Using diet and exercise, you can lower your blood sugar levels.

Maintain a healthy meal plan: Maintaining a healthy meal plan is crucial for managing blood sugar levels. A balanced diet that includes a range of foods, such as lean proteins, whole grains, fruits, and vegetables, is crucial. To create a customized meal plan that suits their particular requirements, pregnant women with gestational diabetes may need to engage with a licensed dietitian.

Watch your consumption of carbohydrates: Since carbohydrates may alter blood sugar levels, it's important to keep an eye on your intake. Women who have gestational diabetes during pregnancy may need to restrict their consumption of carbohydrates to maintain stable blood sugar levels.

Select foods with a low GI: The slower rate of digestion of low-glycemic index meals may aid in blood sugar regulation. Whole grains, fruits, and vegetables are some examples of low-glycemic index foods.

Exercise frequently: Regular exercise may help keep blood sugar levels under control. Before beginning an exercise program, it's crucial to speak with a healthcare professional and make pregnancy-safe exercise choices. Exercises that are often safe for pregnant women include walking, swimming, and yoga.

Regularly check blood sugar levels: Pregnant women with gestational diabetes should do so as directed by a licensed dietician or healthcare professional. This may assist in finding any problems and enable any necessary changes to the diet or exercise regimen.

Water is important to consume in large quantities since it helps to regulate blood sugar levels. Choosing water or other low-sugar drinks over sugary beverages can help you keep hydrated throughout pregnancy.

Get adequate sleep: Sleep is crucial for maintaining blood sugar management and general health. Aim for at least 7-8 hours of sleep each night if you have gestational diabetes and are pregnant.

Manage stress: Because stress may impact blood sugar levels, it's important to do so when pregnant. This can include putting relaxing methods like yoga, meditation, or deep breathing into practice.

Taking medicine as directed may be important in certain circumstances to regulate blood sugar levels. Pregnant women with gestational diabetes should follow their doctor's instructions for taking any prescription medications.

For the best health of the mother and the unborn child, it is crucial to regulate blood sugar levels throughout pregnancy. Pregnant women with gestational diabetes can help control their blood sugar levels and lower the risk of complications from the condition by following a healthy meal plan, monitoring carbohydrate intake, choosing low-glycemic index foods, exercising frequently, monitoring blood sugar levels, drinking plenty of water, getting enough sleep, managing stress, and taking medication as directed.

Medication Options

"High blood sugar levels happen because of hormonal changes that make the body more resistant to insulin in certain pregnant women,

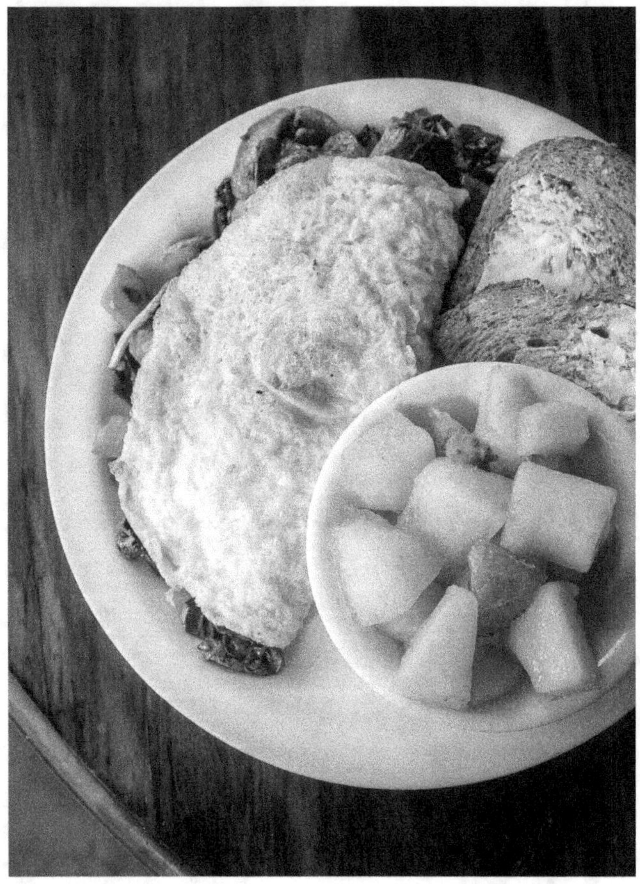

a disease known as gestational diabetes. Medication may be required to regulate blood sugar levels if dietary modifications and exercise are insufficient. It's crucial for ladies with gestational diabetes to comprehend their treatment choices and any possible pregnancy-related side effects.

Insulin is one of the most often used drugs to treat gestational diabetes. Injections of insulin improve the body's ability to metabolize glucose, which helps control blood sugar levels. Injections of synthetic insulin are required when the body's natural production of the hormone insulin is inadequate to control blood sugar. Depending on each person's blood sugar levels and reaction to the medicine, the amount and timing of insulin injections will change.

Gestational diabetes may also be treated with oral medicines like metformin and glyburide. These drugs function by improving insulin sensitivity and decreasing the liver's ability to produce glucose. They have been shown to have fewer negative effects than insulin injections and are usually thought to be safe to use during pregnancy. The individual's blood sugar levels will, however, determine the amount and timing of these drugs, just as they do with insulin.

When taking medication, it's crucial for pregnant women with gestational diabetes to constantly check their blood sugar levels.

This is commonly accomplished by doing routine blood glucose tests at home using a glucose meter. Depending on a number of variables, including gestational age and any preexisting medical issues, the healthcare professional will determine the target blood glucose levels for each woman.

Pregnant women who have gestational diabetes should be informed of any dangers connected to taking medications. Low blood sugar levels may result from insulin injections and induce symptoms including disorientation, lightheadedness, and even fainting. Nausea, vomiting, and diarrhea are examples of adverse effects that oral drugs may produce. The use of medications during pregnancy carries a slight risk of birth abnormalities as well.

It is crucial to go through the possible advantages and disadvantages of pharmaceutical usage with your healthcare professional. To be sure there are no possible conflicts between the medicine recommended for gestational diabetes and any other prescriptions, including over-the-counter vitamins, women should let their healthcare practitioner know about all of the medications they are taking.

Dietary modifications and exercise may help regulate blood sugar levels during pregnancy in addition to medication. An ideal diet for pregnant women with gestational diabetes should include lean proteins, whole grains, fruits, vegetables, and healthy fats. They need to stay away from meals that are heavy in sugar and processed carbs. Blood sugar levels may also be regulated with regular activity such as walking or swimming.

In summary, medication may be a useful therapy choice for pregnant women with gestational diabetes who are unable to manage their blood sugar levels with dietary adjustments and exercise. Commonly recommended treatments include oral drugs like glyburide and metformin as well as insulin injections, each of which has its own potential advantages and disadvantages. In order to monitor blood sugar levels and choose the best treatment strategy, women with gestational diabetes should engage closely with their healthcare professionals. In order to control their blood sugar levels and advance general health while pregnant, ladies should also continue to adhere to a balanced diet and exercise regimen.

Chapter 9

Gestational Diabetes and Postpartum Care

Diabetes of this kind, known as gestational diabetes, affects pregnant women. It may raise the chance of a number of issues during and after pregnancy. Even after giving delivery, women with gestational diabetes need to maintain their blood sugar levels and take care of their health. Women with gestational diabetes need postpartum care in order to avoid further health issues.

Regular visits to the doctor are part of postpartum care, which is intended to make sure that new mothers are healing properly. Women who have gestational diabetes should get this treatment in particular since they run the risk of subsequently acquiring type 2 diabetes. In the ten to twenty years after delivery, women who have had gestational diabetes have a 35–60% probability of getting type 2 diabetes, according to the American Diabetes Association.

Blood sugar level monitoring is one of the most crucial components of postpartum therapy for mothers with gestational diabetes. To ascertain if they have acquired diabetes after giving birth, women may need to do routine at-home blood sugar checks or submit to an oral glucose tolerance test. In order to control their blood sugar levels and lessen their chance of acquiring type 2 diabetes, women may also need to keep up their good eating and activity habits.

Attending follow-up meetings with their healthcare professionals is crucial for pregnant women with gestational diabetes. In addition to screens for other medical concerns like high blood pressure and high cholesterol, these sessions could also include blood tests to check blood sugar levels. The treatment of other health issues, such as controlling weight and mental health, may also be covered by healthcare practitioners.

Women with gestational diabetes should get postpartum care that includes assistance for breastfeeding in addition to medical attention. Breastfeeding may aid women in controlling their blood sugar levels and lower their risk of type 2 diabetes. Healthcare professionals may give advice on how to breastfeed properly and assist you through any difficulties that may occur.

To treat the emotional and psychological effects of the illness, women with gestational diabetes may also profit from support groups or therapy. Due to their diagnosis, women may feel guilty, anxious, or depressed, but these feelings may be managed with support from medical professionals and other women who have had gestational diabetes.

In conclusion, postpartum care is essential for mothers who have gestational diabetes to avoid long-term health issues. Women should continue to keep an eye on their blood sugar levels, maintain a balanced diet and exercise regimen, see their doctors for follow-up visits, get assistance with breastfeeding, and deal with any emotional or psychological issues brought on by their diagnosis. These actions may help women keep their health and well-being at their highest levels while lowering their risk of type 2 diabetes.

The risk of type 2 diabetes after pregnancy.

Gestational diabetes is a transient type of disease that develops during pregnancy and often goes away after giving birth. But women who have experienced gestational diabetes are more likely to eventually acquire type 2 diabetes. The risk of acquiring type 2 diabetes is seven times higher for women with a history of gestational diabetes than it is for women without such a history, according to the Centers for Disease Control and Prevention (CDC).

The risk of developing type 2 diabetes after pregnancy is influenced by several factors, including weight gain during pregnancy, family history of diabetes, age at pregnancy, and ethnicity. Women who are overweight or obese before pregnancy, gain excessive weight during pregnancy, or have a family history of diabetes are at a higher risk of developing type 2 diabetes after pregnancy.

The development of type 2 diabetes after gestational diabetes is a gradual process. The cells in the body become resistant to insulin, the hormone that regulates blood sugar levels, leading to high blood sugar levels. This condition is known as insulin resistance, and it can go on for years before progressing to type 2 diabetes. It is important to note that not all women who have had gestational diabetes will develop type 2 diabetes, but the risk is higher compared to women who did not have gestational diabetes.

The importance of postpartum care for women with gestational diabetes cannot be overstated. Women who have had gestational diabetes should undergo regular follow-up testing to monitor their blood sugar levels and assess their risk of developing type 2 diabetes. The American Diabetes Association recommends that women who have had gestational diabetes undergo a diabetes screening test at least every three years after childbirth.

Apart from regular diabetes screening, women with a history of gestational diabetes can reduce their risk of developing type 2 diabetes by making lifestyle changes. Eating a healthy diet, engaging in regular physical activity, and maintaining a healthy weight are important steps that can reduce the risk of developing type 2 diabetes. These lifestyle changes are particularly important for women who have had gestational diabetes, as they are at a higher risk of developing type 2 diabetes.

In addition to lifestyle changes, medication may also be prescribed to reduce the risk of developing type 2 diabetes. Metformin, a medication used to treat type 2 diabetes, has been shown to be effective in reducing the risk of developing type 2 diabetes in women with a history of gestational diabetes. However, medication should not be seen as a substitute for lifestyle changes but rather as a complementary treatment.

In conclusion, women with a history of gestational diabetes are at a higher risk of developing type 2 diabetes after pregnancy. However, regular diabetes screening, lifestyle changes, and medication, if prescribed, can help reduce the risk of developing type 2 diabetes. It is important for women who have had gestational diabetes to undergo regular follow-up testing and make lifestyle changes to maintain their health and reduce their risk of developing type 2 diabetes.

Recommendations for ongoing management of blood sugar levels.

Gestational diabetes is a temporary condition that usually resolves after childbirth. However, women with gestational diabetes have a higher risk of developing type 2 diabetes later in life. Therefore, ongoing management of blood sugar levels is essential to prevent the development of type 2 diabetes.

The first step in ongoing management is regular blood sugar monitoring. Women who had gestational diabetes should have their blood sugar levels checked regularly, especially during routine health check-ups. This is important to ensure that their blood sugar levels are within the normal range and to identify any changes that may indicate the development of type 2 diabetes.

In addition to regular blood sugar monitoring, women with a history of gestational diabetes should adopt healthy lifestyle habits that can help maintain healthy blood sugar levels. This includes healthy eating habits, regular exercise, and weight management.

Healthy eating habits are crucial in the ongoing management of blood sugar levels. Women with a history of gestational diabetes should continue to follow a healthy and balanced diet that includes whole grains, fruits, vegetables, lean proteins, and healthy fats. They should also avoid high-sugar and high-fat foods and limit their intake of processed foods.

Regular exercise is also important in maintaining healthy blood sugar levels. Women with a history of gestational diabetes should aim for at least 150 minutes of moderate-intensity exercise per week. This can include activities such as brisk walking, cycling, swimming, or dancing. Exercise not only helps regulate blood sugar levels but also promotes weight management and overall health.

Weight management is also important in the ongoing management of blood sugar levels. Women who had gestational diabetes should aim for a healthy weight and maintain a healthy body mass index (BMI). This can be achieved through healthy eating habits and regular exercise.

If lifestyle changes alone are not enough to maintain healthy blood sugar levels, medication may be necessary. In some cases, women with a history of gestational diabetes may need to take medication such as metformin to regulate their blood sugar levels. It is important to work with a healthcare provider to determine the best course of action and to monitor blood sugar levels regularly while on medication.

In conclusion, ongoing management of blood sugar levels is crucial for women with a history of gestational diabetes to prevent the development of type 2 diabetes later in life. This involves regular blood sugar monitoring, healthy lifestyle habits, including healthy eating habits, regular exercise, weight management, and in some cases, medication. It is important to work with a healthcare provider to develop an individualized management plan and to monitor blood sugar levels regularly.

Chapter 10

Conclusion

Final thoughts and words of inspiration.

Many pregnant women may find it difficult to control their gestational diabetes. But it is possible to effectively control blood sugar levels and have a safe pregnancy if you have the necessary tools, resources, and support. To control your blood sugar levels, lead a healthy lifestyle, and consume balanced food, it's crucial to work closely with your medical team.

It's important to keep in mind that each woman's experience with gestational diabetes is different, and what works for one woman may not work for another. In your attempts to control your blood sugar, be persistent and patient, and don't be embarrassed to ask for assistance or support when you need it.

During pregnancy, managing blood sugar levels and promoting general health may be accomplished by including wholesome meals such as whole grains, lean meats, fruits, vegetables, and healthy fats. Making educated food decisions requires using skills like portion management, knowledge of glycemic index and glycemic load, and reading product labels.

For some women, managing blood sugar levels may also require taking medication in addition to diet and exercise. You and your medical team must explore pharmaceutical choices and abide by their advice.

Women with gestational diabetes must also get postpartum treatment. It is crucial to maintain monitoring blood sugar levels and adopt a healthy lifestyle after giving birth for women who have had gestational diabetes since they are at an increased risk of acquiring type 2 diabetes in the future.

Overall, it's important to approach gestational diabetes with optimism and dedication to make good decisions for both you and your unborn child. Gestational diabetes patients may enjoy a healthy pregnancy and a positive postpartum period with the correct services and care.

Additional tools and assistance for treating gestational diabetes

Although managing gestational diabetes might be difficult, it's vital to keep in mind that you're not alone. To assist you on your journey, a wealth of resources and assistance are accessible. Here are some more tools and websites that might help you manage gestational diabetes:

Registered dietician: A registered dietician can provide you with personalized nutritional guidance and assistance to assist you in controlling your blood sugar levels. Additionally, they may provide you with advice on how to plan meals, make appropriate food selections, and manage portions.

Certified Diabetes Educator: A healthcare practitioner with certification in diabetes education is a certified diabetes educator. They may provide you with information about administering insulin, monitoring your blood sugar levels, and other elements of managing diabetes.

Support groups: You might find a feeling of belonging and support by joining a group for women with gestational diabetes. You may impart your knowledge, solicit suggestions and counsel from others, and gain insight from their achievements and setbacks.

Online resources: You may find a wide variety of informational and supportive materials online to help you manage gestational diabetes. The National Institute of Diabetes and Digestive and

Kidney Diseases (NIDDK) and the American Diabetes Association (ADA) are two trustworthy sources.

Exercise regimens: Exercise on a regular basis may help regulate blood sugar levels and enhance general health during pregnancy. Talk to your doctor about safe exercise alternatives, and think about signing up for a pregnant exercise program.

Devices that continuously monitor your blood sugar levels (CGM): CGM devices may provide you with real-time information about your blood sugar levels, which can help you make necessary dietary and activity changes.

Applications for managing diabetes: You can monitor your blood sugar levels, dietary consumption, and exercise routines with a variety of applications for managing diabetes. MySugr, Glucose Buddy, and Diabetes:M are a few well-known applications.

It's crucial to maintain your commitment to your health and well-being since controlling gestational diabetes is a continuous journey. You are capable of effectively controlling your blood sugar levels and having a safe pregnancy with the correct assistance and tools.